Pegan Diet Recipes

The Essential Cookbook For Perfect Looks, Long-Lasting Health And Increased Confidence By Following Easy and Tasty Meals

Cooknest Publishing

__Flynn Davison__

CONTENTS

DRINKS

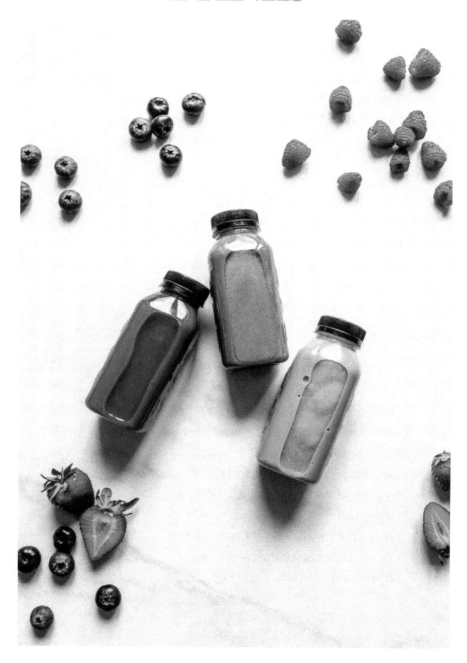

Zero Fat Romaine Lettuce Smoothie

Preparation Time: 15 minutes | Cook time: 0 minutes | Servings 2

1 cup chopped romaine lettuce

2 medium cucumbers, peeled and quartered

1/4 cup chopped mint

1 cup water, divided

1. Place romaine, cucumbers, mint, and 1/2 cup water in a blender and combine thoroughly.

2. Add remaining water while blending until desired texture is achieved.

Nutrition Facts

Calorie 40| Fat 0g| Carbs 9g| Protein 2g

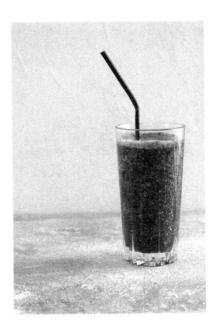

Watercress Mango Smoothie

Preparation Time: 15 minutes | Cook time: 0 minutes | Servings 2

1 cup chopped watercress

1 medium mango, pitted and peeled

1 cup raspberries

11/2 cups oat milk, divided

1. Place watercress, mango, raspberries, and 3/4 cup oat milk in a blender and blend until thoroughly combined.

2. 2 Add remaining oat milk while blending until desired texture is achieved.

Nutrition Facts

Calorie 232| Fat 3g| Carbs 50g| Protein 6g

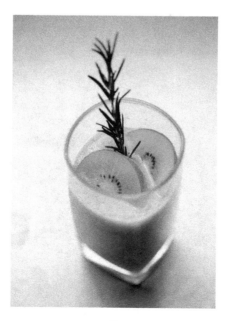

Healthy Watercress Orange Smoothie

Preparation Time: 15 minutes | Cook time: 0 minutes | Servings 2

2 Cup chopped watercress

2 medium oranges, peeled

1 cup strawberries

1 cup blueberries

1 cup water

1 cup canned full-fat coconut milk, divided

1. Place watercress, oranges, strawberries, blueberries, water and 1/2 cup coconut milk in a blender and blend until thoroughly combined.

2. Add remaining coconut milk while blending until desired texture is achieved.

Nutrition Facts

Calorie 310| Fat 15g| Carbs 35g| Protein 4g

Glowing Lettuce Banana Smoothie

Preparation Time: 15 minutes | Cook time: 0 minutes | Servings 3

4 cups chopped romaine lettuce

4 medium pears, cored

1 medium banana, peeled

6 tablespoons lemon juice

2 cups water, divided

1. Place romaine, pears, banana, lemon juice, and 1 cup water in a blender and blend until thoroughly combined.

2. Add remaining water while blending until desired texture is achieved.

Nutrition Facts

Calorie 183| Fat 1g| Carbs 48g| Protein 2g

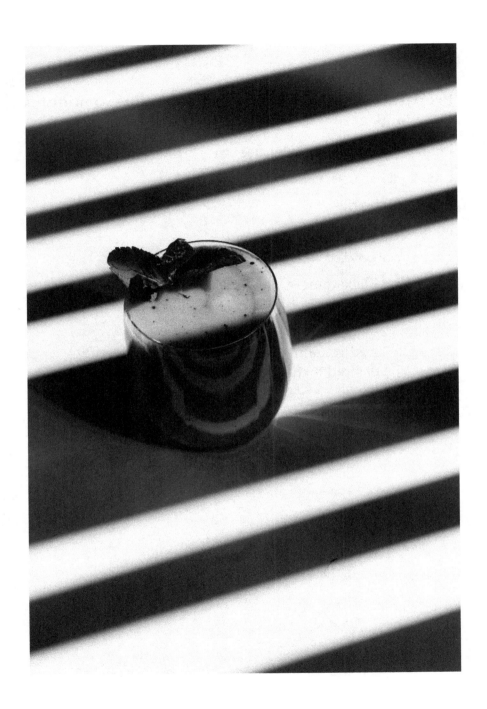

Lettuce & Double Berry Smoothie

Preparation Time: 15 minutes | Cook time: 0 minutes | Servings 2

1 cup chopped romaine lettuce

2 medium bananas, peeled

1 pint strawberries

1 pint blueberries

2 cups unsweetened vanilla almond milk, divided

1. Place romaine, bananas, berries, and 1 cup almond milk in a blender and blend until thoroughly combined.

2. Add remaining almond milk while blending until desired texture is achieved.

Nutrition Facts

Calorie 211| Fat 4g| Carbs 46g| Protein 4g

Vanilla Almond Apple Smoothie

Preparation Time: 15 minutes | Cook time: 0 minutes | Servings 2

2 cups spinach

1 medium banana, peeled

2 medium apples, cored and peeled

2 cups unsweetened vanilla almond milk, divided

1. Place spinach, banana, apples, and 1 cup almond milk in a blender and blend until thoroughly combined.

2. Add remaining almond milk while blending until desired texture is achieved.

Nutrition Facts

Calorie 183| Fat 3g| Carbs 39g| Protein 3g

Vanilla flavoured Banana Smoothie

Preparation Time: 15 minutes | Cook time: 0 minutes | Servings 2

1 cup chopped romaine lettuce

2 medium bananas, peeled

1 tablespoon cocoa powder

1/2 teaspoon vanilla bean pulp

2 cups oat milk, divided

1. Place romaine, bananas, cocoa powder, vanilla bean pulp, and 1 cup oat milk in a blender and blend until thoroughly combined.

2. Add remaining oat milk while blending until desired texture is achieved.

Nutrition Facts

Calorie 230| Fat 3g| Carbs 49g| Protein 7g

Watercress Peachy Banana Smoothie

Preparation Time: 15 minutes | Cook time: 0 minutes | Servings 2

1 cup chopped watercress

1 large orange, peeled

1 medium peach, pitted

1 medium banana, peeled

1 cup canned full-fat coconut milk, divided

1. Place watercress, orange, peach, banana, and 1/2 cup coconut milk in a blender and blend until thoroughly combined.

2. Add remaining coconut milk while blending until desired texture is achieved.

Nutrition Facts

Calorie 300| Fat 15g| Carbs 33g| Protein 4g

Feel Clean Banana- Dandelion Detox Smoothie

Preparation Time: 15 minutes | Cook time: 0 minutes | Servings 2

1/2 cup chopped dandelion greens

1/2 cup arugula

2 cups chopped pineapple

1 medium banana, peeled

1 cup water

1 cup canned full-fat coconut milk, divided

1. Place dandelion greens, arugula, and pineapple, banana, water and 1/2 cup coconut milk in a blender and blend until thoroughly combined.

2. Add remaining coconut milk while blending until desired texture is achieved.

Nutrition Facts

Calorie 315| Fat 17g| Carbs38g| Protein 3g

Grapefruit Watercress Super Smoothie

Preparation Time: 15 minutes | Cook time: 0 minutes | Servings 2

1 cup chopped watercress

1 large grapefruit, peeled

2 medium oranges, peeled

1 medium banana, peeled

1 cup water, divided

1. Place watercress, grapefruit, oranges, banana, and 1/2 cup water in a blender and blend until thoroughly combined.

2. Add remaining water while blending until desired texture is achieved.

Nutrition Facts

Calorie 162| Fat 1g| Carbs 41g| Protein 3g

Six Ingredients- Feel Fresh Smoothie

Preparation Time: 15 minutes | Cook time: 0 minutes | Servings 2

1 cup chopped iceberg lettuce

2 medium pears, cored

1 medium banana, peeled

1/2 cup pitted cherries

1/2 teaspoon vanilla bean pulp

2 cups unsweetened vanilla almond milk, divided

1. Place lettuce, pears, banana, cherries, vanilla bean pulp, and 1 cup almond milk in a blender and blend until thoroughly combined.

2. Add remaining almond milk while blending until desired texture is achieved.

Nutrition Facts

Calorie 216| Fat 3g| Carbs 48g| Protein 3g

Vanilla flavoured Oatmeal Smoothie

Preparation Time: 15 minutes | Cook time: 0 minutes | Servings 2

2 tablespoons rolled oats

1 cup chopped watercress

2 medium peaches, pitted

2 medium apples, cored and peeled

2 cups unsweetened vanilla almond milk, divided

1. Place oats, watercress, peaches, apples, and 1 cup almond milk in a blender and blend until thoroughly combined.

2. Add remaining almond milk while blending until desired texture is achieved.

Nutrition Facts

Calorie 198| Fat 4g| Carbs 43g| Protein 4g

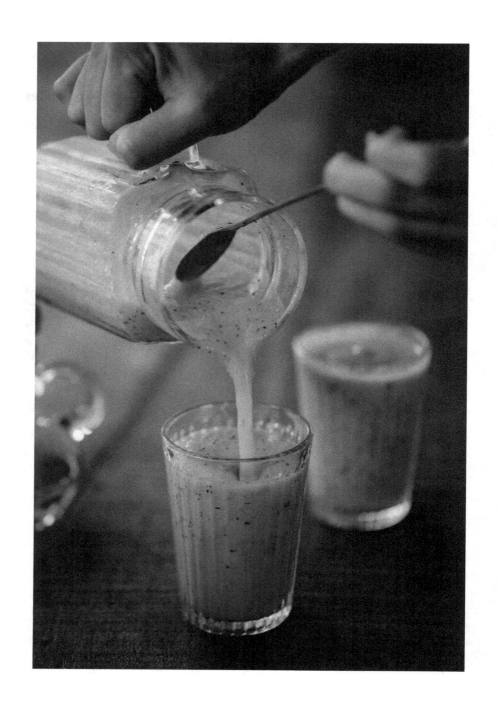

Spinach Zucchini Green Smoothie

Preparation Time: 15 minutes | Cook time: 0 minutes | Servings 2

1 cup spinach

1 medium zucchini, chopped

3 medium carrots, peeled and chopped

2 medium apples, cored and peeled

2 cups water, divided

1. Place spinach, zucchini, carrots, apples, and 1 cup water in a blender and blend until thoroughly combined.

2. Add remaining water while blending until desired texture is achieved.

Nutrition Facts

Calorie 163| Fat 1g| Carbs 40g| Protein 4g

Clear Your Mind Lettuce Smoothie

Preparation Time: 15 minutes | Cook time: 0 minutes | Servings 2

1 cup chopped romaine lettuce

2 medium tomatoes

1 medium zucchini, chopped

2 medium stalks celery, chopped

1 medium cucumber, chopped

1/2 cup chopped green onions

2 cloves garlic, peeled

2 cups water, divided

1. Place romaine, tomatoes, zucchini, celery, cucumber, green onions, garlic, and 1 cup water in a blender and blend until thoroughly combined.

2. Add remaining 1 cup water, if needed, while blending until desired texture is achieved.

Nutrition Facts

Calorie 86| Fat 1g| Carbs 17g| Protein 5g

Feel Fresh Lemony Watercress Smoothie

Preparation Time: 15 minutes | Cook time: 0 minutes | Servings 2

1 cup chopped watercress

1 cup chopped asparagus

1 small lemon, peeled

1 large orange, peeled

1 cup water, divided

1. Place watercress, asparagus, lemon, orange, and $1/2$ cup water in a blender and blend until thoroughly combined.

2. Add remaining water while blending until desired texture is achieved.

Nutrition Facts

Calorie 65| Fat 0g| Carbs 16g| Protein 3g

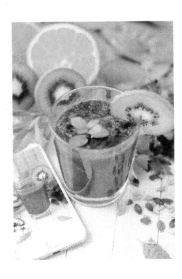

Homemade zucchini Carrot Smoothie

Preparation Time: 15 minutes | Cook time: 0 minutes | Servings 2

1 cup chopped romaine lettuce

1 cup chopped broccoli

1 medium zucchini, chopped

2 medium carrots, peeled and chopped

2 cups water, divided

1. Place romaine, broccoli, zucchini, carrots, and 1 cup water in a blender and blend until thoroughly combined.

2. Add remaining water while blending until desired texture is achieved.

Nutrition Facts

Calorie 71| Fat 1g| Carbs 15g| Protein 4g

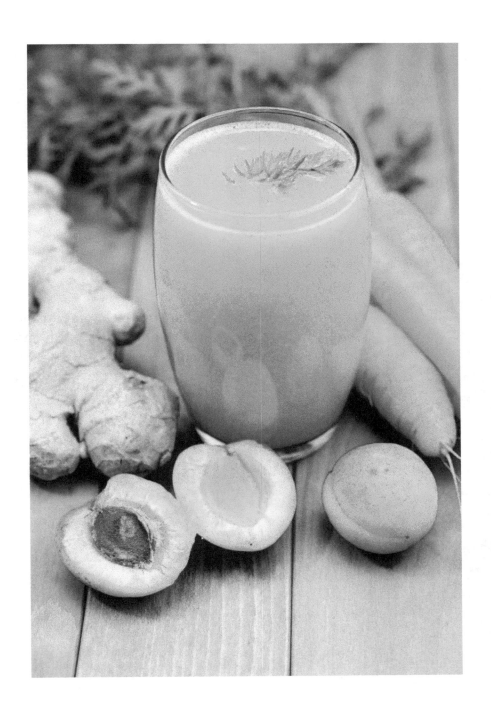

Lemony Grapefruit Watercress Smoothie

Preparation Time: 15 minutes | Cook time: 0 minutes | Servings 2

1 cup chopped watercress

1 large grapefruit, peeled

2 medium oranges, peeled

1 (1/2") piece gingerroot, peeled

1/2 medium lemon, peeled

1 cup water, divided

1. Place watercress, grapefruit, oranges, gingerroot, lemon, and 1/2 cup water in a blender and blend until thoroughly combined.

2. Add remaining water while blending until desired texture is achieved.

Nutrition Facts

Calorie 136| Fat 0g| Carbs 35g| Protein 3g

Apple & Spinach Detox Smoothie

Preparation Time: 15 minutes | Cook time: 0 minutes | Servings 2

1 cup spinach

2 medium green apples, peeled and cored

1/2 medium banana, peeled

1 cup water, divided

1. Place spinach, apples, banana, and 1/2 cup water in a blender and blend until thoroughly combined.

2. Continue adding remaining water while blending until desired texture is achieved

Nutrition Facts

Calorie 241| Fat 1g| Carbs 63g| Protein 2g

Simple Raw Tomato Juice

Preparation Time: 15 minutes | Cook time: 20 minutes | Servings 4

10 large tomatoes, seeded and sliced

1 teaspoon lemon juice

1/4 teaspoon ground black pepper

1 tablespoon maple syrup

1. Place tomatoes in a 2-quart slow cooker and cook on low for 20 minutes.

2. Press cooked tomatoes through a sieve.

3. Add remaining ingredients and chill

Nutrition Facts

Calorie 95| Fat 1g| Carbs 21g| Protein 4g

Four Ingredients Ginger Lemon Water

Preparation Time: 15 minutes | Cook time: 15 minutes | Servings 6

5 cups water

3/4 cup lemon juice

3/4 cup maple syrup

½ piece gingerroot, peeled and sliced

1 Combine all ingredients in a 2-quart or smaller slow cooker.

2 Cover and cook on high for 15 minutes (if mixture begins to boil, turn heat to low).

3 Chill and serve over ice.

4 Remove gingerroot before serving.

Nutrition Facts

Calorie 109| Fat 0g| Carbs 29g| Protein 0g

Detoxifying Spicy Black Tea

Preparation Time: 15 minutes | Cook time: 30 minutes | Servings 22

5 cups water

6 slices fresh ginger

1 teaspoon whole cloves

2 (3") cinnamon sticks

11/2 teaspoons freshly ground nutmeg

1/2 teaspoon ground cardamom

1 cup maple syrup

12 bags black tea

6 cups unsweetened vanilla almond milk

1. Pour water into a 4-quart slow cooker.
2. Put ginger and cloves in a muslin spice bag or a piece of cheese cloth secured with a piece of kitchen twine
3. Add to the cooker along with cinnamon sticks, nutmeg, and cardamom.
4. Cover and cook on low for 15 minutes.
5. Stir in maple syrup until it's dissolved into the water.
6. Add tea bags and almond milk; cover and cook on low for 15 minutes.
7. Remove and discard the spices in the muslin bag or cheesecloth, the cinnamon sticks, and the tea bags.
8. Ladle into teacups or mugs to serve.

Nutrition Facts

Calorie 88| Fat 1g| Carbs 19g| Protein 1g

Sweet Roma Tomato Double Berry Smoothie

Preparation Time: 10 minutes | Cook time: 0 minutes | Servings 3

1 cup sliced strawberries

1 cup raspberries

1 medium Roma tomato, seeded and chopped

1 cup unsweetened rice milk

1 tablespoon maple syrup

1/2 teaspoon vanilla

3 ice cubes

1. Combine all ingredients in a blender and blend until smooth.
2. Pour immediately into glasses and serve.

Nutrition Facts

Calorie 82| Fat 2g| Carbs 18g| Protein 2g

Four Ingredient Healthy Orange water

Preparation Time: 15 minutes | Cook time: 15 minutes | Servings 6

5 cups water

Juice from 5 large oranges

1/2 cup maple syrup

½ piece gingerroot, peeled and sliced

1. Combine all ingredients in a 2-quart slow cooker.

2. Cover and cook on high for 15 minutes (if mixture begins to boil, turn heat to low).

3. Allow cooling and serving chilled. (Remove gingerroot before serving)

Nutrition Facts

Calorie 100| Fat 0g| Carbs 25g| Protein 0g

Herbal Cinnamon Tea

Preparation Time: 15 minutes | Cook time: 5 minutes | Servings 6

4 bags herbal tea

1 teaspoon ground nutmeg

1/2 teaspoon ground cinnamon

1/4 teaspoon ground cloves

5 cups boiling water

1 In a ceramic teapot, combine tea bags and spices.

2 Pour boiling water into teapot.

3 Steep for 5 minutes, then remove tea bags

Nutrition Facts

Calorie 6| Fat 0g| Carbs 0g| Protein0g

Easy Tasty Banana Date Smoothie

Preparation Time: 15 minutes | Cook time: 0 minutes | Servings 2

3 large pitted dates

Water for soaking

3/4 cup unsweetened vanilla almond milk

1 medium banana, peeled

6 ice cubes

1/4 teaspoon vanilla

1. In a small bowl, cover dates with water and soak for at least 10 minutes.

2. Discard soaking water and add dates and all other ingredients to a lender.

3. Process about 1 minute on medium speed until smooth.

Nutrition Facts

Calorie 177| Fat 2g| Carbs 40g| Protein 3g

Sweet and Creamy Banana Apricot Smoothie

Preparation Time: 15 minutes | Cook time: 0 minutes | Servings 2

3 medium apricots, pitted

1 medium banana, peeled

1/2 cup water

1/2 cup canned full-fat coconut milk

4–6 ice cubes

1. Combine all ingredients in a blender and blend until smooth and frosty

Nutrition Facts

Calorie 320| Fat 17g| Carbs 38g| Protein 4g

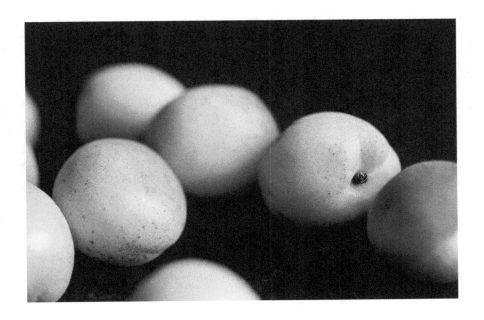

Classic Strawberry Vanilla Almond Smoothie

Preparation Time: 15 minutes | Cook time: 0 minutes | Servings 2

1/2 medium banana, peeled and frozen

1/2 cup frozen strawberries

2 tablespoons ground flaxseed

2 tablespoons rolled oats

1 cup unsweetened vanilla almond milk

1. Place all ingredients in a blender.

2. Purée until smooth.

Nutrition Facts

Calorie 218| Fat 7g| Carbs 35g| Protein 7g

Healthy Frozen Coconut Smoothie

Preparation Time: 15 minutes | Cook time: 0 minutes | Servings 2

11/2 cups mashed and softened coconut meat

1 cup chopped pineapple

1/2 cup chopped mango

1 medium clementine, peeled

2 cups unsweetened almond milk

2 cups ice, divided

1. Combine coconut, pineapple, mango, clementine, and almond milk in a blender with 1/2 cup ice, and blend until thoroughly combined.

2. Add remaining ice gradually while blending until desired consistency is reached.

Nutrition Facts

Calorie 416| Fat 30g| Carbs 38g| Protein 5g

Natural Vanilla Avocado Smoothie

Preparation Time: 15 minutes | Cook time: 0 minutes | Servings 2

1 large ripe avocado, pitted and peeled

1 cup unsweetened vanilla almond milk

1/2 cup water

2 tablespoons maple syrup

3–4 ice cubes

1. Combine all ingredients in a blender and blend until smooth.
2. Serve chilled.

Nutrition Facts

Calorie 365| Fat 24g| Carbs 39g| Protein 4g

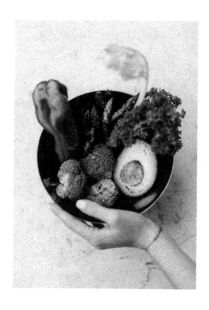

Spinach Tomato Blast Smoothie

Preparation Time: 15 minutes | Cook time: 0 minutes | Servings 2

1 cup spinach

1 medium tomato

1 medium stalk celery, chopped

2 tablespoons cilantro

1 clove garlic, peeled

2 cups water, divided

1. Place spinach, tomato, celery, cilantro, garlic, and 1 cup water in a blender and blend until thoroughly combined.

2. Add remaining 1 cup water while blending until desired texture is achieved.

Nutrition Facts

Calorie 51| Fat 1g| Carbs 10g| Protein 3g

Coconut Milk Shake with Cocoa Nibs

Preparation Time: 15 minutes | Cook time: 0 minutes | Servings 2

1/3 cup canned full-fat coconut milk

2/3 cup water

1/4 cup cacao nibs

1 tablespoon honey

1/2 teaspoon cinnamon

1/4 teaspoon nutmeg

4–6 ice cubes

1. Combine all ingredients in a blender and purée until smooth.

Nutrition Facts

Calorie 365| Fat 25g| Carbs 27g| Protein 5g

Homemade Lettuce Carrot Smoothie

Preparation Time: 15 minutes | Cook time: 0 minutes | Servings 2

2 cups chopped romaine lettuce

3 medium carrots, peeled and chopped

1 medium apple, peeled and cored

1 cup water

1. Combine all ingredients except water in a blender.

2. Add water slowly while blending until desired texture is achieved.

Nutrition Facts

Calorie 93| Fat 1g| Carbs 23g| Protein 2g

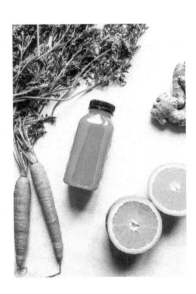

Avocado Nutmeg Oat Milk Smoothie

Preparation Time: 15 minutes | Cook time: 0 minutes | Servings 2

1 cup frozen blueberries

1/2 medium avocado, peeled and pitted

1 cup oat milk

1 cup spinach

1/8 teaspoon ground nutmeg

4–6 ice cubes

1. Combine all ingredients in a blender and purée until smooth.

Nutrition Facts

Calorie 367| Fat 14g| Carbs 59g| Protein 8g

Chilled Three Pears - Banana Smoothie

Preparation Time: 15 minutes | Cook time: 0 minutes | Servings 2

3 medium pears, peeled, cored, and sliced

1 banana, peeled

1 cup unsweetened vanilla almond milk

1 teaspoon cinnamon

2 cups ice, divided

1 Preheat oven to 375°F.

2 Layer pears in a shallow baking dish.

3 Add enough water to cover the bottom of the baking dish, and bake for 20 minutes or until pears are fork tender.

4 Combine pears, banana, almond milk, and cinnamon in a blender with 1/2 cup ice and blend until thoroughly combined.

5 Add remaining ice gradually while blending until desired consistency is reached.

Nutrition Facts

Calorie 215| Fat 2g| Carbs 53g| Protein 2g

Very Cherry Banana Smoothie

Preparation Time: 15 minutes | Cook time: 0 minutes | Servings 2

2 cups pitted cherries

1 medium banana, peeled

1 cup kale

Pulp of 1 vanilla bean

1 cup unsweetened vanilla almond milk

1 teaspoon vanilla extract

1 cup ice, divided

1 Combine cherries, banana, kale, vanilla bean pulp, almond milk, and vanilla extract in the blender with 1/2 cup ice and blend until thoroughly combined.

2 Add remaining ice gradually while blending until desired consistency is reached.

Nutrition Facts

Calorie 170| Fat 2g| Carbs 38g| Protein 3g

Tasty Banana Mango Fruit Drink

Preparation Time: 15 minutes | Cook time: 0 minutes | Servings 2

1 cup chopped mango

1 large banana, peeled

1 cup unsweetened vanilla almond milk

2 cups ice, divided

1 Combine mango, banana, and almond milk in a blender with 1/2 cup ice and blend until thoroughly combined.

2 Add remaining ice gradually while blending until desired consistency is reached.

Nutrition Facts

Calorie 132| Fat 2g| Carbs 30g| Protein 2g

Beets and Carrot Smoothie

Preparation Time: 15 minutes | Cook time: 0 minutes | Servings 2

1 cup chopped beet greens

2 medium beets, peeled and chopped

2 medium carrots, peeled and chopped

1 medium cucumber, peeled and chopped

2 cups water, divided

1 Place beet greens, beets, carrots, cucumber, and 1 cup water in a blender and blend until thoroughly combined.

2 Add remaining 1 cup water while blending until desired texture is achieved.

Nutrition Facts

Calorie 87| Fat 1g| Carbs 20g| Protein 3g

Vegan Vanilla Cashew Smoothie

Preparation Time: 15 minutes | Cook time: 0 minutes | Servings 2

1 cup raw cashews

Water for soaking

Additional 4 cups water for milk

1/2 teaspoon salt

1/2 teaspoon vanilla

1 In a large bowl, cover nuts with plenty of water and allow soaking for at least 1 hour or overnight. Drain.

2 Blend soaked nuts with 4 cups water in a food processor. Purée on high until smooth.

3 Strain through cheesecloth or a sieve. Stir in salt and vanilla.

Nutrition Facts

Calorie 143| Fat 11g| Carbs 8g| Protein 5g

SALADS & DRESSINGS

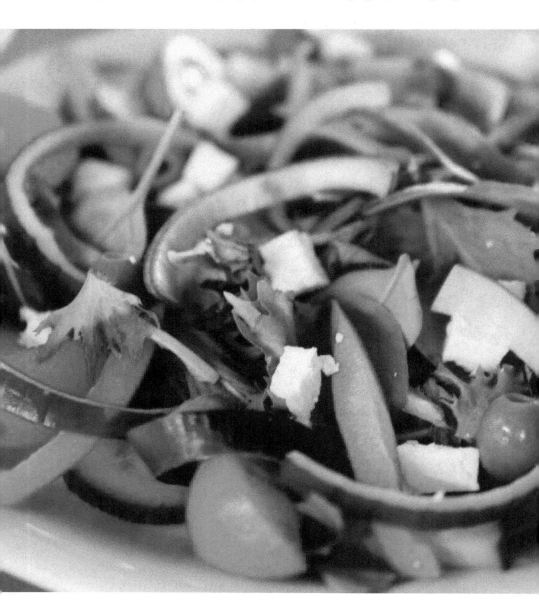

Instant Cantaloupe Blueberry Salad

Preparation Time: 15 minute | Cook time: 0 minute | Servings 4

11/2 cups cubed cantaloupe

1 cup cubed seedless watermelon

1 cup halved green grapes

3/4 cup blueberries

1 tablespoon minced mint leaves

1 teaspoon minced flat-leaf parsley

1. In a large salad bowl, gently toss cantaloupe, watermelon, grapes, and blueberries together.

2. Add mint and parsley to salad. Toss to combine.

3. Serve immediately or chill for up to 2 hours before serving.

Nutrition Facts

Calorie 79| Fats 0g| Carbs 18g| Protein 3g

Paleo Baby Greens & Raspberries Goat Cheese Salad

Preparation Time: 15 minute | Cook time: 30 minute | Servings 4

4 tablespoons lime juice

4 tablespoons olive oil

1/4 teaspoon ground cumin

2 teaspoons minced jalapeño pepper

4 cups mixed baby greens

2 cups raspberries

1/4 cup peeled, thinly sliced red onion

1 ounce crumbled goat cheese

1. Place lime juice, olive oil, cumin, and jalapeño in a blender and blend until smooth.

2. In a large bowl, toss dressing with greens, berries, and onions. Top with goat cheese and serve immediately.

Nutrition Facts

Calorie 184| Fats 15g| Carbs 11g| Protein 3g

Sweet & Spicy Mango Cantaloupe Salad

Preparation Time: 15 minute | Cook time: 15 minute | Servings 4

2 tablespoons mango juice

1 tablespoon walnut oil

1/8 teaspoon chili powder

1/8 teaspoon sweet Hungarian paprika

1/8 teaspoon ground red pepper

3 cups cubed cantaloupe

1/2 cup peeled, diced red onion

1. Whisk mango juice, oil, chili powder, paprika, and red pepper together in a small bowl until oil is emulsified.

2. Place cantaloupe and red onion in a large bowl. Pour dressing over salad and toss well to coat.

3. Cover salad and chill in refrigerator for 15 minutes. Remove bowl from refrigerator, toss gently, and serve.

Nutrition Facts

Calorie 83| Fats 4g| Carbs 13g| Protein 1g

Milky Watermelon Salad

Preparation Time: 15 minute | Cook time: 0 minute | Servings 6

2 tablespoons lemon juice

2 tablespoons maple syrup

2 tablespoons canned full-fat coconut milk

2 tablespoons chopped fresh mint

1/8 teaspoon salt

3 cups cubed cantaloupe

3 cups cubed watermelon

2 cups cubed honeydew melon

1. In large serving bowl, combine lemon juice, maple syrup, coconut milk, mint, and salt and mix well.

2. Add melons and stir gently to coat.

3. Serve immediately, or cover and chill for up to 6 hours before serving.

Nutrition Facts

Calorie 92| Fats 1g| Carbs 221g| Protein 2g

Homemade Peppercorn Vegetable Stock

Preparation Time: 15 minute | Cook time: 30 minute | Servings 4

2 pounds yellow onions, peeled and roughly chopped

1 pound carrots, peeled and roughly chopped

1 pound celery, roughly chopped

11/2 gallons water

1 cup chopped parsley stems

4 sprigs fresh thyme

2 bay leaves

15 peppercorns

1. Place onions, carrots, celery, and water in a large stockpot over medium heat; bring to a simmer and cook, uncovered, for 25 minutes.

2. Add parsley stems, thyme, bay leaves, and peppercorns, and continue to simmer, uncovered, for 5 minutes.

3. Remove from heat and strain stock. Discard solids. Stock can be refrigerated for two to four days or frozen for up to three months.

Nutrition Facts

Calorie 40| Fats 0g| Carbs 9g| Protein 1g

Garlicky Vegetable Stock

Preparation Time: 15 minute | Cook time: 30 minute | Servings 4

3 medium carrots, peeled and coarsely chopped

3 medium parsnips, peeled and coarsely chopped

3 large onions, peeled and quartered

3 whole medium turnips

3 medium rutabagas, quartered

3 medium bell peppers, seeded and halved

2 medium shallots, peeled

1 medium head garlic

1 medium bunch fresh thyme

1 medium bunch parsley

5 quarts water

1. Preheat oven to 425°F. Line a 9" × 13" baking pan with parchment paper. Arrange all the vegetables and herbs in the pan and roast for 15 minutes or until browned. Flip vegetables halfway through.

2. Add vegetables to a 6-quart slow cooker.

3. Add 5 quarts water and cover.

4. Cook on low for 15 minutes

5. Strain stock, discarding the solids. Freeze or refrigerate stock and use within one to two weeks.

Nutrition Facts

Calorie 64| Fats 0g| Carbs 15g| Protein 2g

Rich Garlic Thyme Mushroom Stock

Preparation Time: 15 minute | Cook time: 30 minute | Servings 4

1 quart water

12 ounces white mushrooms

6 parsley stems (with leaves)

1 large onion, peeled and sliced

1 large leek (white part only)

1 medium stalk celery, sliced

2 ounces dried shiitake mushrooms

1 tablespoon minced garlic

11/2 teaspoons black peppercorns

3/4 teaspoon dried sage

3/4 teaspoon dried thyme leaves

1/2 teaspoon ground black pepper

1. Combine all ingredients except ground pepper in a 6-quart slow cooker; cover and cook on low for 30 minutes.

2. Strain, discarding solids; season with ground pepper.

3. Serve immediately, refrigerate and use within one to two weeks, or freeze up to several months.

Nutrition Facts

Calorie 46| Fats 0g| Carbs 9g| Protein 2g

Healthy Cumin Cauliflower Soup

Preparation Time: 15 minute | Cook time: 30 minute | Servings 4

1 pound cauliflower florets

1 (14-ounce) can cannellini beans, drained and rinsed

21/2 cups water

1 medium onion, peeled and minced

2 cloves garlic, peeled and minced

3 teaspoons curry powder

1/4 teaspoon cumin

1. Place all ingredients in a 4-quart slow cooker. Stir. Cook on low for 30 minutes.

2. Use an immersion blender to purée the soup or blend the soup in batches in a blender until smooth.

Nutrition Facts

Calorie 110| Fats 1g| Carbs 20g| Protein 7g

Almond Tomato Onion Soup

Preparation Time: 15 minute | Cook time: 20 minute | Servings 4

4 cups chopped tomatoes

1/2 cup peeled, chopped onion

4 whole cloves

2 cups Basic Vegetable Stock

2 tablespoons olive oil

2 tablespoons almond flour

Juice from 1 medium lime

1. In a stockpot, combine tomatoes, onion, cloves, and vegetable stock over medium-high heat. Bring to a boil, reduce heat to medium-low, and simmer for about 20 minutes.

2. Remove from heat and strain into a large bowl. Discard solids.

3. In the now-empty stockpot, combine olive oil and almond flour. Stir until mixture thickens.

4. Gradually whisk in tomato mixture and stir in lime juice.

Nutrition Facts

Calorie 144| Fats 9g| Carbs 15g| Protein 3g

Easy Spicy Zucchini Coconut Milk Soup

Preparation Time: 15 minute | Cook time: 25 minute | Servings 8

4 cups sliced, peeled zucchini

4 cups Basic Vegetable Stock

4 cloves garlic, peeled and minced

2 tablespoons lime juice

2 teaspoons curry powder

1 teaspoon dried marjoram leaves

1/4 teaspoon celery seeds

1/2 cup canned full-fat coconut milk

1/4 teaspoon cayenne pepper

1 teaspoon paprika

1. Combine all ingredients except coconut milk, cayenne pepper, and paprika in a 4–6-quart slow cooker, and cook on high for 25 minutes

2. Process zucchini mixture with coconut milk in a blender until combined.

3. Season with cayenne pepper. Sprinkle with paprika and serve warm.

Nutrition Facts

Calorie 58| Fats 3g| Carbs 8g| Protein 2g

Mushroom Thyme and Celery Soup

Preparation Time: 15 minute | Cook time: 25 minute | Servings 6

2 tablespoons olive oil

1 medium shallot, peeled and finely minced

1 (8-ounce) package cremini mushrooms, sliced

1 medium bunch celery, trimmed and thinly sliced

6 cups Basic Vegetable Stock

1 teaspoon dried thyme leaves

1 teaspoon salt

1/8 teaspoon ground white pepper

1 tablespoon lemon juice

1. In large pot, heat olive oil over medium heat. Add shallot; cook until softened, about 3 minutes.

2. Add mushrooms; cook and stir until mushrooms give up their liquid, about 8 minutes.

3. Add celery and cook for 4 minutes longer.

4. Add stock, thyme, salt, and white pepper, and bring to a simmer.

5. Cover pot, reduce heat to low, and simmer for 15–20 minutes or until soup is blended. Stir in lemon juice and serve immediately.

Nutrition Facts

Calorie 100| Fats 5g| Carbs 13g| Protein 3g

Kale Pesto Almond Soup

Preparation Time: 15 minute | Cook time: 15 minute | Servings 6

3 tablespoons olive oil

1 medium onion, peeled and chopped

2 cloves garlic, peeled and minced

1 medium jalapeño pepper, seeded and minced

3 tablespoons almond flour

1 teaspoon ground cumin

5 cups Basic Vegetable Stock

2/3 cup almond butter

1/3 cup unsweetened almond milk

1/2 teaspoon salt

1/8 teaspoon ground black pepper

2/3 cup sliced almonds, toasted

1/2 cup Kale Pesto

1. In large soup pot, heat olive oil over medium heat.

2. Add onion, garlic, and jalapeño; cook and stir for 5 minutes.

3. Add almond flour and cumin; cook for 1 minute. Then beat in stock and simmer for 2 minutes until thickened.

4. Add almond butter, almond milk, salt, and black pepper. Simmer for 10 minutes until flavors are blended.

5. In a small bowl combine almonds with Kale Pesto and mix.

6. Serve soup with this mixture for topping.

Nutrition Facts

Calorie 396| Fats 33g| Carbs 20g| Protein 11g

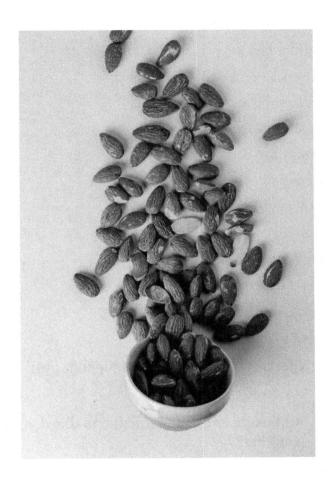

Authentic Lemony Tomato Soup

Preparation Time: 15 minute | Cook time: 0 minute | Servings 6

1 (28-ounce) can chopped tomatoes

1 medium green bell pepper, seeded and chopped

3 medium tomatoes, peeled and chopped

1 large cucumber, peeled and chopped

1 small onion, peeled and chopped

2 tablespoons olive oil

1/2 teaspoon ground black pepper

1/2 teaspoon paprika

1/4 teaspoon cayenne pepper

1 teaspoon chopped chives

2 teaspoons chopped parsley

1/2 clove garlic, peeled and minced

41/2 teaspoons lemon juice

1. Blend canned tomatoes in blender until smooth.
2. Pour into a large bowl.
3. Add remaining ingredients to bowl and stir to combine.

1. Refrigerate at least 12 hours. Serve chilled.

Nutrition Facts

Calorie 90| Fats 5g| Carbs 11g| Protein 2g

Coriander Squash Coconut Soup

Preparation Time: 15 minute | Cook time: 30 minute | Servings 6

2 cups Roasted Vegetable Stock

2 medium acorn squash, peeled, seeded, and cut into cubes

1/2 cup peeled, chopped onion

1/2 teaspoon ground cinnamon

1/4 teaspoon ground coriander

1/4 teaspoon ground cumin

1/2 cup canned full-fat coconut milk

1 tablespoon lemon juice

1 teaspoon ground black pepper

2. Combine stock, squash, onion, cinnamon, coriander, and cumin in a 4-quart slow cooker.

3. Cover and cook on high for 30 minutes.

4. Blend squash mixture, coconut milk, and lemon juice in a food processor until smooth.

5. Season with pepper before serving.

Nutrition Facts

Calorie 117| Fats 3g| Carbs 22g| Protein 2g

Squash Cinnamon Butternut Soup

Preparation Time: 15 minute | Cook time: 5 minute | Servings 4

1 tablespoon olive oil

1 medium onion, peeled and chopped

1 pound butternut squash, peeled, seeded, and chopped

1/2 cup ground flaxseed

32 ounces Basic Vegetable Stock (see recipe in this chapter)

1 cup unsweetened almond milk

1/2 teaspoon ground cinnamon

1/4 teaspoon ground cloves

1/4 teaspoon ground nutmeg

1. In a large soup pot or Dutch oven, heat olive oil over medium-high heat.

2. Sauté onion and butternut squash in oil for 5 minutes.

3. Add ground flaxseed and stock and bring to a boil over high heat. Reduce heat to low and simmer for 25 minutes.

4. In batches, purée squash mixture in blender or food processor and return to pot.

5. Stir in almond milk, cinnamon, cloves, and nutmeg.

Nutrition Facts

Calorie 215| Fats 10g| Carbs 28g| Protein 7g

Sweet and Toasted Pumpkin Soup

Preparation Time: 15 minute | Cook time: 30 minute | Servings 6

1 medium sugar pumpkin, peeled, seeded, and chopped (reserve seeds)

1/4 teaspoon salt

3 medium leeks, sliced

11/2 teaspoons minced fresh ginger

2 tablespoons olive oil, divided

1/2 teaspoon grated lemon zest

1 teaspoon lemon juice

2 quarts Basic Vegetable Stock

1 teaspoon ground black pepper

1. Preheat oven to 375°F.

2. Clean pumpkin seeds thoroughly, place them on a baking sheet, and sprinkle with salt to taste. Roast for approximately 5–8 minutes, until light golden. Remove from oven and set aside.

3. Place chopped pumpkin in a large baking dish with leeks, ginger, and 1 tablespoon olive oil; roast for 20 minutes or until tender.

4. Transfer the cooked pumpkin mixture to a large stockpot and add zest, juice, stock, and black pepper. Bring to a boil over medium-high heat. Reduce heat to low and simmer for 10 minutes.

5. To serve, ladle into serving bowls.

6. Drizzle with remaining olive oil and sprinkle with toasted pumpkin seeds.

Nutrition Facts

Calorie 141| Fats 5g| Carbs 23g| Protein 3g

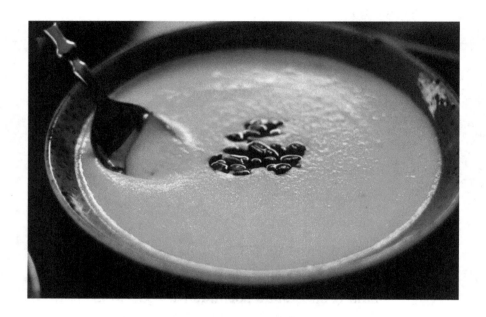

Creamy Sweet Potato Mango Soup

Preparation Time: 15 minute | Cook time: 30 minute | Servings 4

3 large sweet potatoes, peeled and cubed

2 cups Roasted Vegetable Stock

1 (15-ounce) can sliced mangoes, untrained

1/4 teaspoon ground allspice

1/2 cup canned full-fat coconut milk

1. Place all ingredients except coconut milk in a 4-quart slow cooker.

2. Cover and cook on low for 30 minutes.

3. When sweet potatoes are soft, purée soup in a blender and stir in coconut milk.

Nutrition Facts

Calorie 230| Fats 5g| Carbs 45g| Protein 4g

Guava Strawberries & Peach Soup

Preparation Time: 15 minute | Cook time: 30 minute | Servings 4

2 cups cubed cantaloupe

2 cups cubed peaches

11/2 cups guava nectar

2 tablespoons fresh lime juice

1 cup sliced strawberries

1. Combine cantaloupe, peaches, guava nectar, and lime juice in a blender or food processor and purée until smooth. Chill.

2. To serve, spoon soup into individual bowls and garnish with strawberry slices.

Nutrition Facts

Calorie 146| Fats 1g| Carbs 36g| Protein 2g

Tender Vegetables Soup

Preparation Time: 15 minute | Cook time: 10 minute | Servings 4

1 large head cauliflower, chopped

3 large stalks celery, chopped

1 medium carrot, peeled and chopped

2 cloves garlic, peeled and minced

1 medium onion, peeled and chopped

2 teaspoons ground cumin

1/2 teaspoon ground black pepper

1 tablespoon chopped parsley

1/4 teaspoon dill

1. In a large soup pot or Dutch oven, combine cauliflower, celery, carrot, garlic, onion, cumin, and black pepper.

2. Add water to just cover ingredients in pot. Bring to a boil over high heat.

3. Reduce heat to low. Simmer about 8 minutes or until vegetables are tender.

4. Stir in parsley and dill before serving.

Nutrition Facts

Calorie 62| Fats 1g| Carbs 13g| Protein 4g

SIDE DISHES

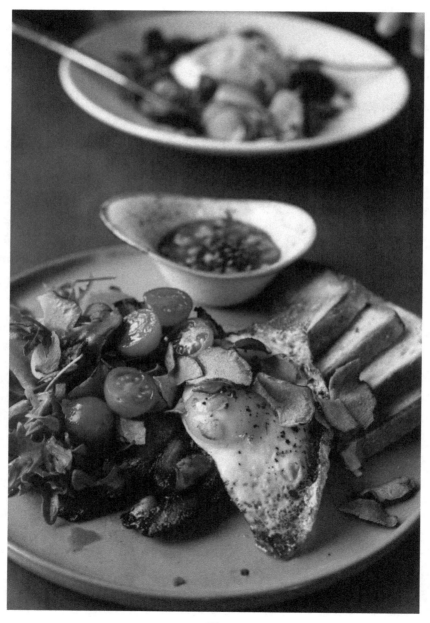

Easy and Healthy Fried Cauliflower

Preparation Time: 10 minutes | Cook time: 10 minutes | Servings 4

1 head fresh cauliflower, greens removed, washed

1 tablespoon coconut oil or extra-virgin olive oil

Salt, to taste

Freshly ground black pepper, to taste

1. Break the cauliflower into florets, put in a food processor, and pulse in 1-second intervals 10 to 15 times, until the cauliflower resembles rice.

2. Alternately, grate the florets using the medium-size slots of a box grater.

3. Heat the coconut oil in a large skillet over medium heat until melted.

4. Add the cauliflower, cover, and cook until softened and the odour dissipates, 5 to 8 minutes.

5. Remove the lid, season with salt and pepper, and fluff with a fork.

Greens with Lemon wedges

Preparation Time: 5 minutes | Cook time: 10 minutes | Servings 2

1 large bunch (1 pound) Swiss or rainbow chard

1 large lemon

2 tablespoons extra-virgin olive oil

½ medium red onion, minced

¼ teaspoon salt

¼ teaspoons freshly ground black pepper

1. Leaves from 1 small bunch fresh herbs (parsley, cilantro, basil, or dill), minced (optional)

2. Rinse and lightly pat dry the chard (a little water helps them steam faster).

3. Slice the stems into ½-inch pieces and set aside. Tear the leafy greens into 3-inch pieces and set aside.

4. Using a zester or the fine side of a box grater, grate the lemon and set the zest aside. Cut the lemon into wedges and set aside.

5. Heat the olive oil in a large skillet or Dutch oven over medium heat.

6. When it is hot, add onion and chard stems and cook, stirring occasionally, until soft and translucent, 2 to 4 minutes.

7. Add the greens, cover, and steam until just wilted, about 1 minute. Remove the lid, add the reserved lemon zest, salt, pepper, and herbs (if using).

8. Toss to combine.

9. Serve the greens with the lemon wedges for squeezing just before enjoying.

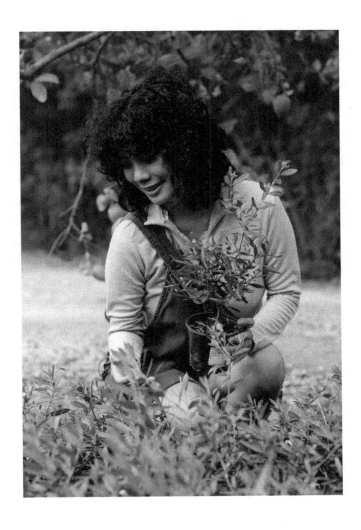

Homemade Portabella Mushroom Green Stir Fry

Preparation Time: 5 minutes | Cook time: 15 minutes | Servings 2

10 ounces cremini or baby portabella mushrooms

2 tablespoons extra-virgin olive oil

¼ teaspoon salt

¼ teaspoons freshly ground black pepper

4 cups baby greens (spinach, kale, or a mix)

1 tablespoon chopped fresh rosemary

1. Clean any dirt off of the mushrooms with a paper towel. Cut the mushrooms into ½-inch-thick slices.

2. Heat the olive oil in a large skillet over medium-high heat.

3. When it is hot, add the mushrooms in a single layer and cook, not stirring or flipping, until browned on one side, about 2 minutes.

4. Flip the mushrooms and cook until browned on the other side, about 2 minutes.

5. Reduce the heat to medium and continue to cook until the mushrooms have released their juices and are tender, another 5 to 8 minutes.

6. Season with the salt and pepper.

7. Add the baby greens, cover, and cook until just wilted, 30 to 60 seconds. Stir in the rosemary and serve.

Pepper Roasted Squash

Preparation Time: 10 minutes | Cook time: 30 minutes | Servings 2

2 medium delicate squash (about 2 pounds)

1 tablespoon extra-virgin olive oil

1 tablespoon maple syrup

¼ teaspoon salt

¼ teaspoon freshly ground black pepper

1. Preheat the oven to 425°F.

2. Slice each squash lengthwise in half. Scoop out the seeds. Flip the squash, cut-side down, and slice into 1-inch pieces.

3. Place the squash on a baking sheet and toss with the olive oil and maple syrup until evenly coated.

4. Spread out the squash in a single layer so the pieces do not overlap.

5. Roast until tender and browned, flipping once halfway, 20 to 25 minutes.

6. Season with the salt and peppers.

Sweet Paprika Fry with Chopped Dill

Preparation Time: 20 minutes | Cook time: 20 minutes | Servings 2

2 large sweet potatoes (¾ pound total), peeled

1 tablespoon extra-virgin olive oil or melted coconut oil

½ teaspoon salt

¼ teaspoons freshly ground black pepper

½ teaspoon paprika (regular or smoked)

3 tablespoons chopped fresh dill (optional)

1. Preheat the oven to 425°F. Line a baking sheet with aluminum foil or parchment paper.

2. Slice the sweet potatoes lengthwise in half and then into ¼-by-¼-inch matchsticks, adding them to a large bowl of cold water to soak for a few minutes while prepping

3. Drain and dry thoroughly with paper towels.

4. Place the potatoes on the prepared baking sheet.

5. Toss with the oil and spread out in a single layer so the fries are not overlapping or touching.

6. Turn all the pieces to point in the same direction.

7. Bake for 15 minutes, remove from the oven, and flip the fries using a flat metal spatula.

8. Make sure the fries are not overlapping or touching and are facing the same direction.

9. Return to the oven and bake until the fries are browned and cooked through, another 15 minutes.

10. Turn off the oven, prop open the door, and allow the fries to cool and crisp up for 10 minutes.

11. Remove from the oven and season with the salt, pepper, and paprika (if using). Toss to coat, sprinkle with the dill (if using), and enjoy.

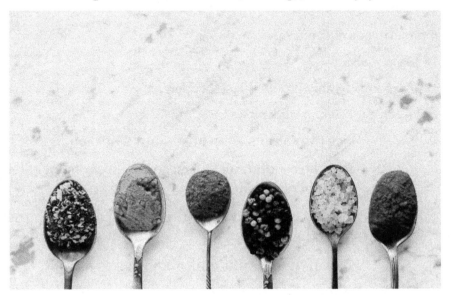

Tender Carrot Coconut Curry

Preparation Time: 3 minutes | Cook time: 15 minutes | Servings

1 pound carrots, peeled

3 tablespoons coconut oil

¼ teaspoon salt

¼ teaspoons freshly ground black pepper

1 cup full-fat coconut milk or water

1. Slice the carrots at an angle into 2½-inch pieces.

2. Heat the coconut oil in a large Dutch oven or skillet over medium heat.

3. Add the carrots and turn to coat; season with the salt and pepper.

4. Pour in the coconut milk and bring to a boil.

5. Reduce the heat to a simmer, cover, and cook until the carrots are just tender, 7 to 10 minutes.

6. Remove the lid, increase the heat, and continue to cook until the water fully evaporates, then serve.

Seasonal Vegetable Mix

Preparation Time: 10 minutes | Cook time: 10 minutes | Servings 4

2 tablespoons extra-virgin olive oil

1 small onion, chopped

1 small eggplant, unpeeled, cut into ½-inch cubes

1 large red bell pepper, seeded and cut into ½-inch pieces

1 large zucchini, cut into ½-inch cubes

6 to 8 ripe tomatoes cut into ½-inch pieces, reserving the juices

¼ cup packed fresh basil leaves, chopped

¼ teaspoon salt

¼ teaspoons freshly ground black pepper

1. Heat the olive oil in a large, deep skillet or Dutch oven over medium heat.

2. Add the onion and eggplant and cook, stirring occasionally, until the onion is slightly browned and the eggplant is tender, about 5 minutes.

3. Add the bell pepper and zucchini and cook, stirring occasionally, until tender, about 10 minutes.

4. Stir in the tomatoes and their juices, cover, and simmer until the vegetables are tender and the ratatouille thickens, 5 minutes.

5. Remove the lid, stir in the basil, and season with the salt and pepper.

6. Serve warm or cover and chill for at least 1 hour or up to overnight to serve cold; this allows the flavors to meld.

Onion Black pepper Corn Salad

Preparation Time: 15 minutes | Cook time: 0 minutes | Makes 2 cup

1 large red onion, diced into ½-inch pieces

2 cups apple cider vinegar

1 teaspoon salt

1 tablespoon whole black peppercorns

1. In a large glass jar or bowl with a lid, add the onions, vinegar, salt, and pepper. Give the mixture a quick stir.

2. Cover and refrigerate overnight. The onions will keep in the refrigerator for about 3 weeks.

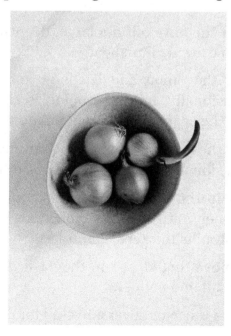

Tomato & Onion Egg Stir Fry

Preparation Time: 15 minutes | Cook time: 10 minutes | Servings 3

2 tablespoons avocado oil, or as needed

6 eggs, beaten

4 ripe tomatoes, sliced into wedges

2 green onions, thinly sliced

1. Heat 1 tablespoon avocado oil in a wok or skillet over medium heat.

2. Cook and stir eggs in the hot oil until mostly cooked through, about 1 minute.

3. Transfer eggs to a plate.

4. Pour remaining 1 tablespoon avocado oil into wok

5. Cook and stir tomatoes until liquid has mostly evaporated, about 2 minutes.

6. Return eggs to wok and add green onions

7. Stir until eggs are fully cooked, about 5 minutes.

Scrambled Pepper Egg

Preparation Time: 5 minutes | Cook time: 10 minutes | Servings 2

¼ cup vegetable oil

1 teaspoon ground turmeric

1 teaspoon ground coriander

Salt to taste

½ cup finely chopped onion

3 green Chile peppers, sliced

2 large eggs

1. Heat oil in a skillet over medium heat; add turmeric, coriander, and salt.

2. Cook and stir onion and green Chile peppers in the seasoned oil until onion is slightly tender, about 5 minutes.

3. Crack eggs into the skillet and season with salt

4. Cook and stir until eggs are set and scrambled, about 5 minutes.

Five Spiced Beef Stew with Potato and Zucchini

Preparation Time: 15 minutes | Cook time: 30 minutes | Servings 8

½ pound beef for stew, such as beef chuck roast, cut into 1-inch chunks

3 tablespoons olive oil

2 (3 inch) pieces fresh ginger root, peeled and diced

3 cloves garlic, minced

2 onions, peeled and diced

2 celery ribs, chopped

2 tablespoons curry powder, or to taste

2 teaspoons coriander powder

1 teaspoon Asian five-spice powder

1 teaspoon ground turmeric

2 carrots, peeled and sliced

Parsnips, peeled and sliced

2 potatoes, peeled and cubed

1 zucchini, sliced

2 apples - peeled, cored and chopped

1 cup raisins

1 cup cashews

½ cup water

1. Preheat oven to 350 degrees F (175 degrees C). Line a roasting pan with aluminum foil.

2. Meanwhile, heat the olive oil in a deep pot over medium-high heat.

3. Stir in the ginger, garlic, onions, and celery, and cook until vegetables soften, about 5 minutes.

4. Mix in the curry powder, coriander powder, five-spice powder, and turmeric, and toss to evenly coat the onion mixture.

5. Cook about 5 minutes more, and stir in the carrots, parsnips, potatoes, zucchini, and apples.

6. Stir in the beef with its cooking liquid, raisins, and cashews, and toss to evenly blend the spices.

7. Pour the beef and vegetable mixture into the prepared roasting pan. Drizzle 1/2 cup water over the mixture. Cover the pan with aluminum foil.

8. Bake in preheated oven until heated through, about 20 minutes

Spicy Beef and Tomato Coconut Curry

Preparation Time: 15 minutes | Cook time: 30 minutes | Servings 6

2 tablespoons ghee (clarified butter)

2 cloves garlic, crushed

1 large onion, finely sliced

2 Serrano peppers, thinly sliced

2 whole cloves, bruised

1 teaspoon garam masala

1 teaspoon ground coriander

½ teaspoon Chile powder

1 teaspoon turmeric

1 ½ teaspoons ground cumin

1 ½ pounds beef tenderloin, cubed

1 teaspoon salt

1 cup chopped tomatoes

⅔ Cup coconut milk

1 (10 ounce) bag spinach

1 teaspoon lemon juice

1. Heat the ghee in a large saucepan over medium heat.

2. Stir in the garlic and onion, and cook until softened, about 5 minutes.

3. Add the Serrano, and continue to cook for another 1 minute.

4. Season with the cloves, garam masala, and coriander, Chile powder, turmeric, and cumin, cook for 2 to 3 more minutes to release the flavor.

5. Stir in the beef and salt, cook for 1 minute more.

6. Add the tomatoes, coconut milk, and spinach.

7. Bring to a simmer, then cover, and cook for 10 minutes, stirring occasionally.

8. Uncover, then stir in the lemon juice, and cook for 2 more minutes, stirring frequently, until the sauce has thickened.

Cashew Prawns with Tender Vegetables

Preparation Time: 15 minutes | Cook time: 20 minutes | Servings 8

2 ¼ pounds peeled and deveined medium shrimp

¼ teaspoon turmeric powder

¼ teaspoon ground red pepper

3 tablespoons cashews

5 whole cardamom pods, broken

2 (3 inch) cinnamon sticks

1 teaspoon whole black peppercorns

4 teaspoons sunflower oil

½ red onion, diced

½ teaspoon garlic paste

¾ teaspoon ginger paste

salt to taste

½ teaspoon garam masala

1 large bay leaf

½ cup diced roma tomatoes

2 green bell peppers, seeded and diced

1 (14 ounce) can coconut milk

1. Season the shrimp with turmeric powder and Chile powder, and set aside.

2. Toast the cashews, cardamom, cinnamon, and peppercorns in a skillet over medium heat until toasted and fragrant, about 7 minutes; remove from the skillet and set aside

3. Heat the sunflower oil in a large skillet over medium-high heat.

4. Add the onion, garlic, and ginger; cook and stir until the onion has softened and begun to lose its red color, about 5 minutes.

5. Stir in the shrimp and toasted spice mixture along with the salt, garam masala, bay leaf, tomatoes, and green pepper.

6. Cook and stir until half of the shrimp has begun to turn pink, then pour in the coconut milk, cover, and bring to a simmer.

7. Cover, and reduce heat to medium-low.

8. Simmer until the shrimp are opaque and the vegetables are tender, about 5 minutes.

Chickpea Carrots Mix with Yogurt Gravy

Preparation Time: 15 minutes | Cook time: 30 minutes | Servings 6

4 sun-dried tomatoes, chopped

½ teaspoon mustard seeds

¼ teaspoon cardamom seeds

1 teaspoon ghee (clarified butter), or as needed

2 teaspoons onion, chopped

1 teaspoon sliced ginger

1 clove garlic, chopped

1 teaspoon garam masala

1 teaspoon turmeric

½ teaspoon ground cinnamon

½ teaspoon ground cloves

1 (15 ounce) can chickpeas, drained

2 small carrots, sliced

1 Chile pepper, chopped

½ cup whole-milk yogurt, at room temperature

½ cup vegetable broth, or as needed (Optional)

1. Place sun-dried tomatoes in a bowl and cover with boiling water. Let soak until softened, about 10 minutes. Drain.

2. Crush mustard seeds and cardamom seeds using a mortar and pestle. Heat ghee in a skillet over medium heat; add crushed spices, onion, ginger, garlic, garam masala, turmeric, cinnamon, and cloves.

3. Fry until mixture is light brown in color, 3 to 5 minutes.

4. Add drained sun-dried tomatoes, chickpeas, carrots, and chile pepper; cook until softened as desired, about 25 minutes.

5. Stir in yogurt. Add broth to thin curry if necessary

SEAFOOD

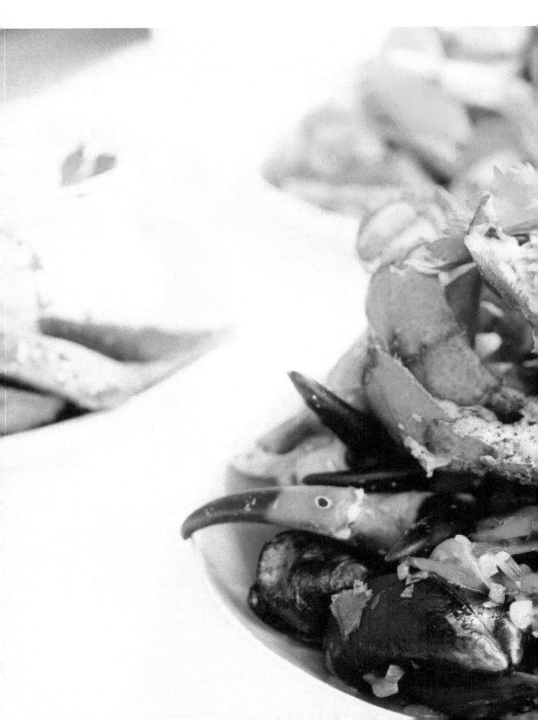

Peppery Shrimp and Steak for Two

Preparation Time: 30 minutes | Cook time: 25 minutes | Servings 2

12 medium shrimp, peeled and deveined

2 filet mignon steaks

2 Teaspoons olive oil

1 Tablespoon butter, melted

1 Tablespoon finely minced onion

1 Teaspoon steak seasoning

1 Tablespoon finely minced onion

1 Tablespoon white wine

1 Teaspoon Worcestershire sauce

1 Teaspoon seafood seasoning

1/8 Teaspoon freshly ground black pepper

1 Teaspoon lemon juice

1 Teaspoon dried parsley

1. In a bowl, whisk 1 Tablespoon olive oil, onion, butter, Worcestershire sauce, wine, lemon juice, parsley, seafood seasoning, garlic, and black pepper together

2. Toss to coat evenly. Cover bowl with plastic wrap and refrigerate for flavors to blend, at least 15 minutes.

3. Preheat an outdoor grill for medium-high heat and lightly oil the grate. Coat steaks with 2 Teaspoons olive oil; sprinkle with steak seasoning.

4. Cook steaks until they are beginning to firm and have reached your desired doneness, 5 to 7 minutes per side.

5. Transfer steaks to a platter and loosely tent with a piece of aluminum foil.

6. Remove shrimp from marinade and grill until they are bright pink on the outside and the meat is no longer transparent in the canter, 2 to 3 minutes per side.

Nutrition Facts

Calorie 444| Fats 34.5g| Carbs 2.7g| Protein 9g

Avocado Nori with Pickled Ginger

Preparation Time: 15 minutes | Cook time: 30 minutes | Servings 2

2 sheets sushi nori

1 medium avocado, pitted and peeled

2 tablespoons sesame seeds, divided (optional)

113 g smoked salmon (about 4 thin slices)

1 medium cucumber, cut into matchsticks

3 Tablespoons pickled ginger (optional)

1 Teaspoon wasabi paste (optional)

Gluten-free soy sauce, tamari, or coconut amino, for dipping

1. Lay 1 piece of nori on a sheet of parchment paper or aluminium foil on a flat surface.

2. In a small bowl, mash the avocado with a fork.

3. Spread half of the avocado mixture on the nori sheet, leaving a ½-inch strip uncovered along the top edge.

4. Sprinkle 1 Tablespoon of the sesame seeds (if using), evenly over the avocado. Arrange 2 pieces of the smoked salmon horizontally, covering the avocado.

5. Arrange the cucumber horizontally, running up the length of the sheet and creating columns to cover the salmon.

6. Wet the tip of your finger and run it along the exposed seam. Roll the nori tightly away from you, using the foil as a guide and pressing firmly to seal.

7. Repeat the process with the remaining nori sheet and ingredients, and refrigerate both for at least 30 minutes to firm up.

8. Using a very sharp or serrated knife, slice each roll into 6 to 8 pieces.

9. Serve with pickled ginger and wasabi (if using) and soy sauce for dipping.

Nutrition Facts

Calorie 487 | Fats 32g| Carbs 26g| Protein 28g

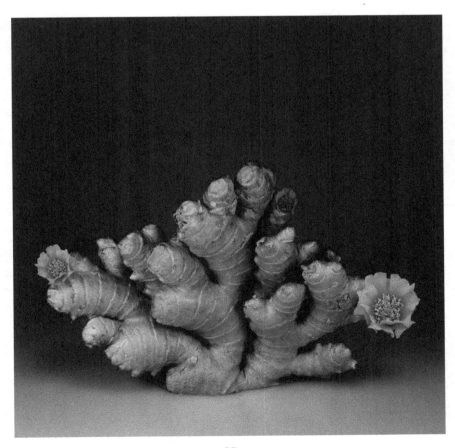

Creamy Salmon Capers with Spiralled Zoodles

Preparation Time: 30 minutes | Cook time: 5 minutes | Servings 2

A small shallot, chopped

1 Tablespoon of almond flour

1 cup sour cream

1/2 cup parmesan

1/3 cup sliced mushrooms of your choice

1 cup broccoli florets

1 Tablespoon capers

1 Tablespoon chopped chives

2 tablespoons s chopped parsley

2 fillets of wild Alaskan salmon

1 Tablespoon avocado oil

3 Tablespoon s pastured butter

2 cloves of garlic, minced

Lemon juice to taste

Black pepper to taste

1. Descale and wash the fish. Fry the salmon with the avocado oil for a few minutes, turning once (do not overcook).

2. Remove its skin and eat it. Add lemon juice on the fish, and set aside.

3. Heat water in a small water and add the mushrooms to boil for a few minutes.

4. Add the broccoli florets for another 1-2 minutes (must remain a little bit crunchy). Strain, set aside.

5. In a large pot heat the butter with the black pepper, garlic and shallot.

6. Add the sour cream and parmesan when browned. Stir to combine, but don't let it get too cooked (no more than 30 seconds on fire, just enough for the parmesan to melt).

7. Cut the salmon in small pieces, add it to the cream.

8. Add the mushrooms, broccoli, and capers, and carefully combine.

9. Sprinkle with chives or parsley; serve with spiralled "zoodles".

Nutrition Facts

Calorie 216.9| Fats 10.9g| Carbs 5.8g| Protein 24g

Garlicky Fish Fillets with Parsley leaves

Preparation Time: 30 minutes | Cook time: 30 minutes | Servings 4

2 skinless Arctic char or other whitefish fillets

1 Teaspoon kosher salt

1 Teaspoon freshly ground black pepper

½ cup extra-virgin olive oil

3 cloves garlic, minced

¾ cup fresh parsley leaves, minced, divided

¼ cup grated lemon zest (from 6 small or 4 large lemons), divided

1. Place the fish fillets lengthwise in a 13-by-9-inch baking dish and season with the salt and pepper on both sides.

2. In a small bowl, whisk together the olive oil, garlic, half of the parsley, and half of the lemon zest. Pour evenly over the fish, cover, and marinate in the refrigerator for at least 30 minutes and up to overnight.

3. Preheat the oven to 350°F. 3. Bake the fish until just cooked through, 15 to 20 minutes.

4. Cut each fillet into 2 pieces, top evenly with the remaining parsley and lemon zest, and serve with Lemony Sautéed Chard with Red Onion and Herbs or another vegetable side or salad.

Nutrition Facts

Calorie 216.9 | Fats 10.9g| Carbs 5.8g| Protein 24g

Best Tuna Grape Salad

Preparation Time: 10 minutes | Cook time: 5 minutes | Servings 4

1/2 stalk of celery

5-6 grapes

1 good quality tuna

1 Tablespoon of mayo

1 Tablespoon Black pepper

1 romaine lettuce

1. Drain the tuna, and place on a bowl. Cut into smaller pieces using your hands.

2. Wash the celery and grapes, and cut them very thinly.

3. Add them to the bowl.

4. Add the mayo, black pepper, and mix well using a spoon.

5. Serve on romaine lettuce leaves, or refrigerate for up to 1 day.

Nutrition Facts

Calorie 170| Fats 7g| Carbs 4g| Protein 20g

Easy Butter Shrimp Scampi with Parsley Leaves

Preparation Time: 15 minutes | Cook time: 10 minutes | Servings 3

454 g jumbo shrimp (about 12), peeled and deveined

3 Tablespoons extra-virgin olive oil, divided

6 cloves garlic, minced

1 cup unsalted chicken broth or stock

Grated zest and juice from

1 medium lemon

½ Teaspoon red pepper flakes, or to taste

¼ Teaspoon sea salt or Himalayan salt, or to taste

½ Teaspoon freshly ground black pepper, or to taste

¼ cup (½ stick) cold unsalted grass-fed butter, cubed

8 cups baby spinach leaves

2 to 3 Tablespoons chopped fresh parsley (optional)

1. Pat the shrimp very dry with paper towels. Heat 2 tablespoons of the olive oil in a large skillet over medium-high heat.

2. Add the shrimp and cook until pink, flipping once, about 2 minutes per side. Transfer to a large bowl or plate. 2

3. Reduce the heat to medium and add remaining 1 Tablespoon oil. Add the garlic and cook until just fragrant, about 1 minute.

4. Add the broth, lemon zest and juice, red pepper flakes, salt, and black pepper, increase the heat to medium-high, and bring to a simmer.

5. Reduce the sauce by half, scraping up any browned bits from the bottom with a wooden spoon, about 5 minutes.

6. Remove the pan from the heat and allow cooling slightly. Add butter, one cube at a time, stirring continually with a wooden spoon until the sauce thickens.

7. To serve, divide spinach evenly among four plates. Top each plate with about 4 shrimp. Divide the sauce evenly among the plates and garnish with the parsley.

Nutrition Facts

Calorie 644 | Fats 46g| Carbs 9g| Protein 53g

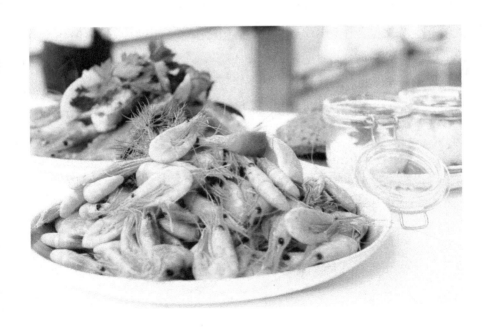

One pan Broiled Salmon with Yellow Miso

Preparation Time: 25 minutes | Cook time: 10 minutes | Servings 2

2 salmon fillets

¼ cup white or yellow miso

2 tablespoons rice or coconut vinegar

2 tablespoons sesame oil, divided

1 Tablespoon gluten-free soy sauce, tamari, or coconut amino

1 Tablespoon minced fresh ginger

1 clove garlic, minced

680 g (medium bunch) baby bok choy, core removed, sliced into 1½-inch pieces, white stem and leafy green parts separated

2 tablespoons thinly sliced scallion whites (optional)

2 tablespoons thinly sliced scallion greens, for garnish (optional)

1. Heat the broiler to high.

2. On a baking sheet or broiler pan, place the salmon, skin-side down, and pat it dry.

3. In a small bowl, whisk together the miso, vinegar, 1 Tablespoon of the sesame oil, the soy sauce, ginger, and garlic.

4. Spread 2 tablespoons of the glaze evenly over the top of the salmon, setting aside the remainder. Let it stand for 10 minutes, if you have time.

5. Broil the salmon until the glaze is bubbly, 3 to 4 minutes. Cover it loosely with foil and continue to broil until slightly pink in the center, another 3 to 4 minutes.

6. Remove the salmon from the broiler, remove the foil, and let it cool.

7. In a large skillet over medium-high heat, heat the remaining 1 Tablespoon sesame oil.

8. Add the bok choy stems and scallion whites (if using) and cook until just tender, 2 to 3 minutes.

9. Stir in the remaining miso glaze and cook until fragrant, 30 to 60 seconds.

10. Add the bok choy greens, cover, and steam until just wilted, 30 seconds. Toss to coat with the sauce.

11. To serve, divide the bok choy evenly between two plates.

12. Top each with a salmon fillet and sprinkle with scallion greens (if using).

Nutrition Facts

Calorie 602| Fats 36g| Carbs 20g| Protein 45g

Garlic and Herb Mussels in Rose Broth

Preparation Time: 18 minutes | Cook time: 10 minutes | Servings 4

32 ounce mussels

1 Tablespoon extra-virgin olive oil

2 shallots, minced

3 cloves garlic, minced

2 cups chicken or Veggie Trimmings Stock

¼ cup lemon juice (from 2 lemons)

¼ cup chopped fresh parsley, plus more for garnish

¼ cup chopped fresh dill (optional)

3 Tablespoons chopped fresh thyme

½ Teaspoon salt

¼ Teaspoon freshly ground black pepper

¼ Teaspoon red pepper flakes (optional)

3 cups baby spinach (or spinach leaves torn into smaller pieces)

2 tablespoons cold unsalted grass-fed butter, cubed

1. Rinse the mussels under cold running water, pulling off their black beards as needed. Place in a strainer to drain and set aside.

2. Heat the oil in a large, deep skillet, stockpot, or Dutch oven over medium-high heat.

3. Add the shallots and cook, stirring, until soft and translucent, about 2 minutes. Add the garlic and cook until fragrant, 30 seconds.

4. Add the stock, lemon juice, herbs, salt, pepper, and red pepper flakes (if using), and stirring to combine. Bring the stock to a boil.

5. Add the mussels, cover, and cook, undisturbed, until the mussels open their shells, about 5 minutes.

6. Reduce the heat to low. Discard any mussels that have not yet opened. Divide the mussels among four large serving bowls.

7. Add the spinach to the broth, cover, and cook until just wilted, 1 to 2 minutes. Remove the lid and turn off the heat. Let sit for 1 minute, then add the cold butter, one piece at a time, stirring in each one until fully melted before adding the next one.

8. Spoon the broth over the mussels in the bowls, garnish with more parsley if you like, and serve.

Nutrition Facts

Calorie 342| Fats 16g| Carbs 17g| Protein 13g

Spicy Crabs with Chilled Coleslaw Mix

Preparation Time: 17 minutes | Cook time: 30 minutes | Servings 2

1 package shredded coleslaw mix

Grated zest and juice of 1 medium lemon

Grated zest of 1 medium navel orange

2 tablespoons Dijon mustard

2 large eggs

1 Tablespoon Dijon mustard

½ Teaspoon sea salt

½ Teaspoon Old Bay seasoning or paprika

¼ Teaspoon freshly ground black pepper

1 can cooked jumbo lump crab meat, drained and patted dry

¾ cup cooled or chilled cooked

Easy Cauliflower Rice, mashed with a fork

2 tablespoons chopped fresh parsley

2 tablespoons extra-virgin olive oil

1. To make the slaw, toss the coleslaw mix with the lemon zest and juice, orange zest, and mustard in a large bowl until evenly coated.

2. Refrigerate it for at least 30 minutes.

3. In a medium bowl, whisk together the eggs, mustard, salt, Old Bay seasoning, and pepper.

4. Fold in the crab, cauliflower rice, and parsley until well combined. Refrigerate until slightly firm, about 10 minutes.

5. Remove the crab mixture from the refrigerator and form into four patties about 2 inches thick and 3 inches in diameter.

6. Heat the olive oil in a large skillet or cast-iron pan over medium-high heat. When the oil is hot, add two of the crab cakes.

7. Cook until golden brown, about 3 minutes per side. Transfer to a paper towel–lined plate. Repeat with the remaining cakes.

8. Place two crab cakes on each plate and serve with the chilled slaw.

Nutrition Facts

Calorie 438| Fats 21g| Carbs 15g| Protein 52g

Coconut Salmon with Scallion Greens

Preparation Time: 10 minute | Cook time: 15 minutes | Servings 2

2 (6-ounce) salmon fillets

¼ cup white or yellow miso

2 tablespoons rice or coconut vinegar

2 tablespoons sesame oil, divided

1 tablespoon gluten-free soy sauce, tamari, or coconut amino

1 tablespoon minced fresh ginger

1 clove garlic, minced

1½ pounds (medium bunch) baby bok choy, core removed, sliced into 1½-inch pieces, white stem and leafy green parts separated

2 tablespoons thinly sliced scallion whites (optional)

2 tablespoons thinly sliced scallion greens, for garnish (optional)

1. Heat the broiler to high.

2. On a baking sheet or broiler pan, place the salmon, skin-side down, and pat it dry.

3. In a small bowl, whisk together the miso, vinegar, 1 tablespoon of the sesame oil, the soy sauce, ginger, and garlic.

4. Spread 2 tablespoons of the glaze evenly over the top of the salmon, setting aside the remainder. Let it stand for 10 minutes, if you have time.

5. Broil the salmon until the glaze is bubbly, 3 to 4 minutes.

6. Cover it loosely with foil and continue to broil until slightly pink in the center, another 3 to 4 minutes.

7. Remove the salmon from the broiler, remove the foil, and let it cool.

8. In a large skillet over medium-high heat, heat the remaining 1 tablespoon sesame oil.

9. Add the bok choy stems and scallion whites (if using) and cook until just tender, 2 to 3 minutes.

10. Stir in the remaining miso glaze and cook until fragrant, 30 to 60 seconds.

11. Add the bok choy greens, cover, and steam until just wilted, 30 seconds. Toss to coat with the sauce.

12. To serve, divide the bok choy evenly between two plates. Top each with a salmon fillet and sprinkle with scallion greens (if using).

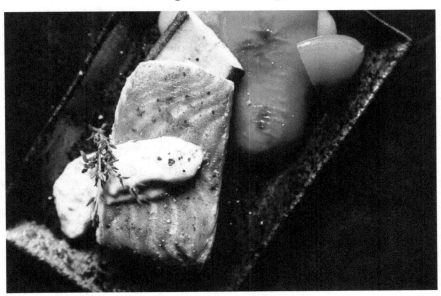

Soy dipped Avocado Sushi Roll

Preparation Time: 15 minute | Cook time: 0 minute | Servings 2

2 sheets sushi nori

1 medium avocado, pitted and peeled

2 tablespoons sesame seeds, divided (optional)

4 ounces smoked salmon (about 4 thin slices)

1 medium cucumber, cut into matchsticks

3 tablespoons pickled ginger (optional)

1 teaspoon wasabi paste (optional)

Gluten-free soy sauce, tamari, or coconut amino, for dipping

1. Lay 1 piece of nori on a sheet of parchment paper or aluminium foil on a flat surface.

2. In a small bowl, mash the avocado with a fork.

3. Spread half of the avocado mixture on the nori sheet, leaving a ½-inch strip uncovered along the top edge.

4. Sprinkle 1 tablespoon of the sesame seeds (if using), evenly over the avocado. Arrange 2 pieces of the smoked salmon horizontally, covering the avocado.

5. Arrange the cucumber horizontally, running up the length of the sheet and creating columns to cover the salmon.

6. Wet the tip of your finger and run it along the exposed seam. Roll the nori tightly away from you, using the foil as a guide and pressing firmly to seal.

7. Repeat the process with the remaining nori sheet and ingredients, and refrigerate both for at least 30 minutes to firm up.

8. Using a very sharp or serrated knife, slice each roll into 6 to 8 pieces. Serve with pickled ginger and wasabi and soy sauce for dipping

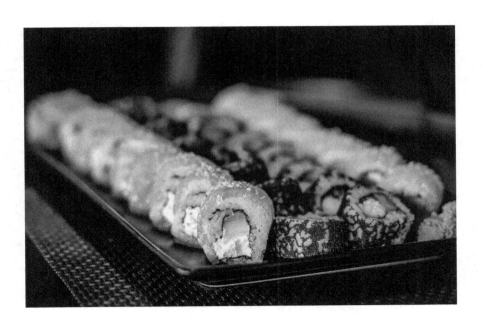